HOMEMADE

MEDICAL FACE
MASK

Self-protection against Infectious diseases, Viral Germs and bacteria with step-by-step Guide making an effective face mask in 15 mins

Caroline Gold K.

Caroline Gold K.

Copyright@2020 by Caroline Gold K.

All rights reserved. No part of this book is should reproduced, stored in a retrieval system, or transmitted in any form or by any means – electronic, mechanical, photocopy, recording, scanning, or other – without a prior written permission of the publisher.

Publisher's Note

The publisher has taken great care to vouch for the accuracy of the information published and to describe generally accepted practices.

The author, editors, and publishers will not be held liable for any error or omitted items or any consequences from the application of the information in this book and make no warranty, expressed concerning the contents of the book.

Table of Contents

Introduction

Face mask belongs to Personal protective equipment (PPE) for protection against the spread of infection or illness or contact from infected an infected person.

It is designed to provide a protective barrier against splashes and droplets impacting the wearer's nose, mouth and respiratory tract. It fits fairly loosely to the user's face..

Face mask are resistant to fluid, can be disposed of after use and have loose-fitting protection devices, which creates a barrier between the mouth and nose parts of the human face and the present environment. Nevertheless, masks do not completely seal face, unlike other types of respirators, and are not reliable in providing the required level of protection from inhaling infectious aerosols.

Unfortunately, due to the recent pandemic outbreak of an acute respiratory disease ravaging many, we can see not only a lack of hand sanitizers and antiseptics but also medical masks.

There is also a severe shortage of N95 masks, which helps protect medical professionals like doctors and nurses from acquiring the disease.

Face mask, which have not yet been proven to effectively block out the tiniest particles that transmit the respiratory disease is also in short supply in stores.

Based on the latest recommendation from the Centers for Disease Control and Prevention's for the people's voluntary use of face coverings in public, in places where the risk of transmitting the acute respiratory diseases from person to person is higher, homemade masks and face coverings can be now be seen as new normal in public places.- from masks with elastic straps to bandana masks.

If you're considering making your face mask, this book will be a guide in the process of making homemade face masks made from fabric materials.

Fabric face masks do not replace medical grade face masks but are now in use in non-critical areas of hospitals.

It is important to note that homemade face masks are not as effective as the CDC recommended **N95 masks**, and cannot serve as a substitute but an alternative as it offers some benefits in addition to following other precautions:

- It prevents large particles from being ejected while coughing or sneezing.
- It offers protection to others when you cough and sneeze if you are infected.
- Encourage mindfulness in behavior, including avoiding touching one's mouth, nose and eyes
- Gives you a sense of protection

What are Face masks?

Face masks are nose and mouth protection tools utilized for preventing the spread of diseases. They are loose-fitting guards with ear loops or ties or bands at the back of the head.

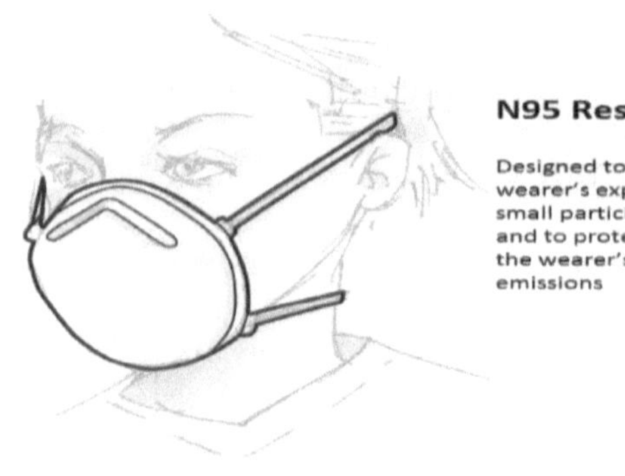

N95 Respirator

Designed to reduce the wearer's exposure to very small particles and droplets and to protect patients from the wearer's respiratory emissions

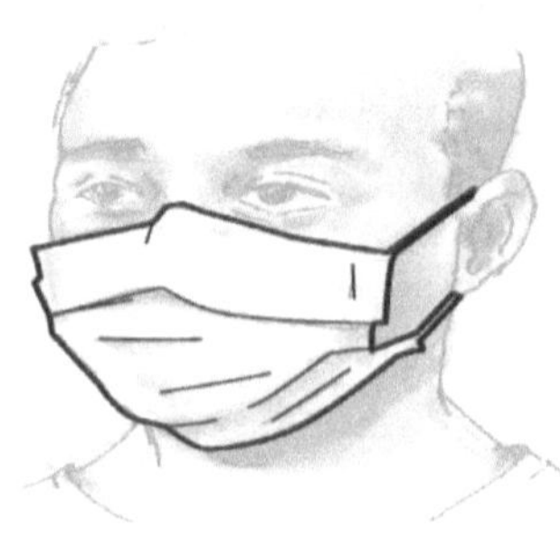

Face/Surgical Mask

Designed to reduce the wearer's exposure to droplets and to protect patients from the wearer's respiratory emissions.

How Face Masks Work

When someone with an Acute Respiratory Disease coughs, sneezes, or talks, they send tiny droplets of the disease into the air.

A face mask will cover your mouth and nose. It will block the release of virus-filled droplets into the air when you cough or sneeze. This helps slow the spread of disease.

When to use a mask

- Wear a mask when and if taking care of an ill person suspected to have the acute respiratory diseases.
- Wear a mask if you have contacted the flu or infected with a respiratory ailment.
- Masks are very effective when combined with other safe hygiene like regular hand-cleaning with alcohol-based hand solution or soap and running water.
- If there is a coughing person in the home.
- Wear a mask when visiting a hospital, clinic, or nursing home.

- If you are taking care of or visiting loved ones who are immune sensitive.
- If it is allergy season to help filter out some allergens.
- If you are spray painting or spraying other types of chemicals.
- If you are cleaning your home or bathroom

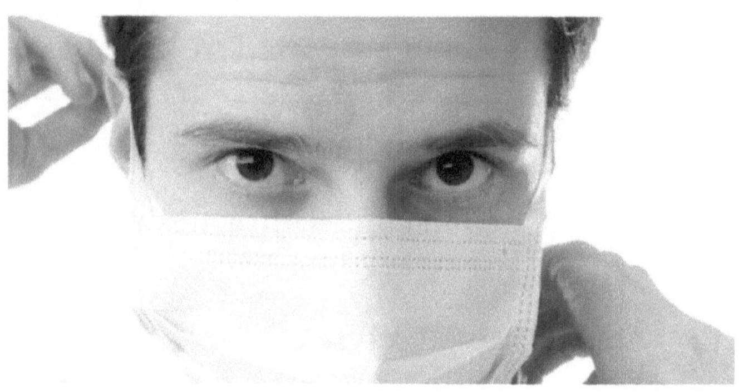

How to put on a face mask

- Before using a face mask, ensure you clean hands with an alcohol-based hand solution or wash for at least 20 seconds with soap and clean water.

- Ensure that nose and mouth protected with no gaps between the face and the mask.
- While the mask is on your face, avoid touching it. Clean your hands with alcohol-based hand rub or soap and water when you accidentally do.
- Replace with a new mask or get soiled and do not reuse.
- After use, remove the mask from behind and do not touch the front of the mask. Discard in a refuse closed bin or burn; clean hands with alcohol-based hand rub or soap and water.

When taking off that mask

- Wash hands thoroughly with an antibacterial hand wash or use sanitizer before taking off the mask.
- Hold mask only by the loops or

- bands only; do not touch the mask itself, as it could be contaminated.
- Carefully remove the mask
- by firstly unhooking or untieing the ear loops or lifting the bottom bands over your head first and the top band next.
- Holding the mask loops, ties, or bands, discard the mask by placing it in a covered trash bin.
- After removing the mask, wash your hands thoroughly or use hand sanitizer.

Requirements for a good face mask

- Comfortably fitted snugly against the side of the face
- Must be secured with ties or ear loops
- Must include multiple layers of fabric

- Allow for breathing without restriction

Materials needed to make a face mask at home

To produce a face mask, these items will come in handy:

- *Cotton fabric:* Face masks should be made from high quality, tightly woven pure cotton material. Other materials that can serve as an alternative are t-Shirts, bandana, handkerchief, pillowcase made from cotton.
- Elastic bands
- A sewing machine kits. You can meet a tailor if you do not know how to sew
- A porous proved yet breathable material to go between the fabric.
- A filtering material, which is incorporated to block smaller particles

- use a double layer of cotton materials a filter

If you do *not have a sewing skill, you can opt for a no-sew face mask* by using a fabric glue and an iron. The iron fuses the fabric and glue tightly and is also used for the creation of pleats when making a thicker mask.

Do not:

- touch the mask once it's secured on your face, as it might have pathogens on it
- dangle the mask from one ear
- hang the mask around your neck
- crisscross the ties
- reuse single-use masks

Importance and benefits in making a homemade face mask

- face masks with fabrics can be made at home from everyday materials in unlimited supply.

- The risk of people without symptoms spreading the respiratory disease through speaking, coughing, or sneezing is minimal.

- Better chances of protection than not using any mask and offer some protection, especially where social distancing is hard to maintain.

QUICK PROTECTION TIPS AGAINST AN EPIDEMIC OR PANDEMIC ACUTE RESPIRATORY DISEASES

Based on the current scientific transmission evidence and action of an epidemic or pandemic acute respiratory disease, the below protection tips should adhere to.

- Take regular showers as a daily routine to prevent respiratory germs that might have stuck on your body when in contact with people gathering in place, some may neglect daily routines, but showering is a must because acute respiratory diseases have an incubation period.

- Keep your clothes clean. Do not wear the same clothes for many days. Do laundry frequently.

- Stop nail-biting, thumb sucking, and rubbing eyes.

- Stop scratching your head, face, or body.

- Wash fruits and vegetables, and avoid eating them immediately in aisles, stores, or car.

- Do not litter the inside and your environment. This activity could increase the risk for household members, while scattering around the community can burden the sanitation workers. Recent instances of people throwing used masks and gloves in public places will increase the risk for

waste management workers and trash
pickers.

- Clean your car. Dispose of leftovers
  and edibles, trash, masks, and gloves.

- Maintain hygiene while growing your
  hair, beard, or nails or using hair and
  face accessories.

- Cover face when sneezing or
  coughing.

- Wash your hands after using
  restrooms, coming back from public
  places, after grocery shopping,
  pumping gas, using elevators, or using
  high traffic doorknobs or electric
  switches.

- Clean your desk space, cell phone, and
  computer devices.

- Do not rely on carryout or delivery as
  your sole source of food for every

meal every day, and be sure to eat enough and consume healthy foods.

- Do not reuse wipes, masks, gloves, and personal care devices without cleaning them.

- Regular intake of fruits and vegetables rich in Vitamin C to boost your immune system

- If you have fever, cough and difficulty breathing, seek medical care early

- Maintain social distancing

- Use a bleach mixture to clean floors

- Clean the floors in your sitting room, kitchen, and bathroom, using a water mixed with a cup of bleach to mop your floors.

- Clean internal surfaces with a disinfectant to kill germs.

Safety tips

- In a public setting, especially in areas of significant community-based transmission like a pharmacy or superstores, wear a face mask

- Do not face masks on children under the age of 2; people with difficulty in breathing, unconscious people , or amputated persons.

- Healthcare professionals should exercise extreme caution when and while using fabric made face masks. The face masks should be used with a face shield that covers the entire sides of the face and extends to the jaw.

Making a DIY Face Mask for the prevention of a Respiratory Disease

Fabric mask with 1/4" Elastic Band

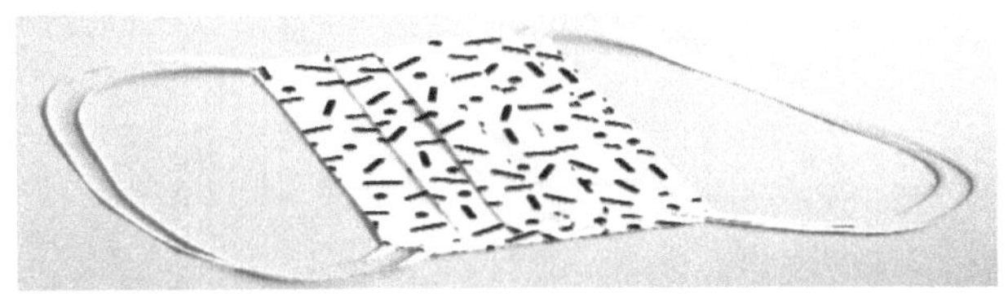

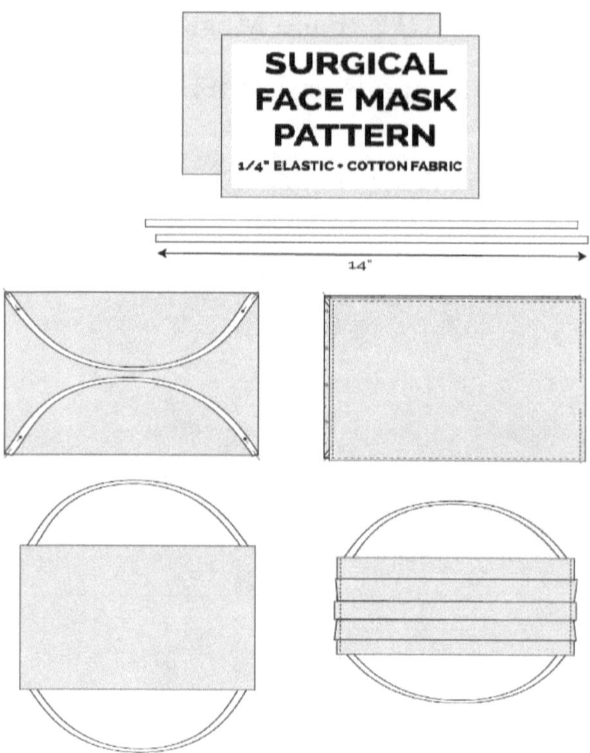

- Measure two lengths of 1/4" elastic 14" band each and cut. Fasten one length of the elastic band with a pin at the top corners of the fabric. Do the same with the length of the elastic at the bottom of the fabric. Place the second fabric material showing the alternate side.

- Sew all edge of the fabric material with seam spacing of about 1.4", leaving a little opening to allow for turning. Now hold the little opening, then turn and create pleats with the iron maintaining the patterns on the material.

- Sew and backstitch the pleats down and close the existing little opening.

Handmade face mask with elastic cording

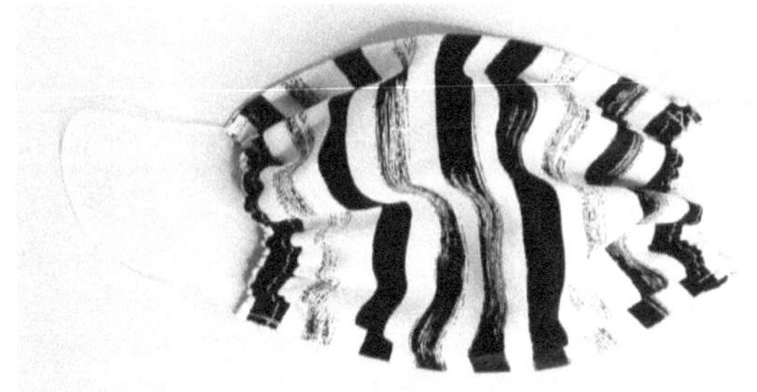

- Cut two squares from the pattern and sew both right sides of the squares with allowing a seam spacing allowance of 1/4" all the way around, while leaving a little opening on one side of the squares.

- Turn the right side of the square out and iron both sides with an allowance o 3/8" and sew together. Use a yarn needle or embroidery needle to thread through the opening, 7 inches around the elastic and tie.

- Spin around the elastic and knot inside the casing, Gather fabric with the elastic band, and sew both top and bottom parts for mask to hold firmly.

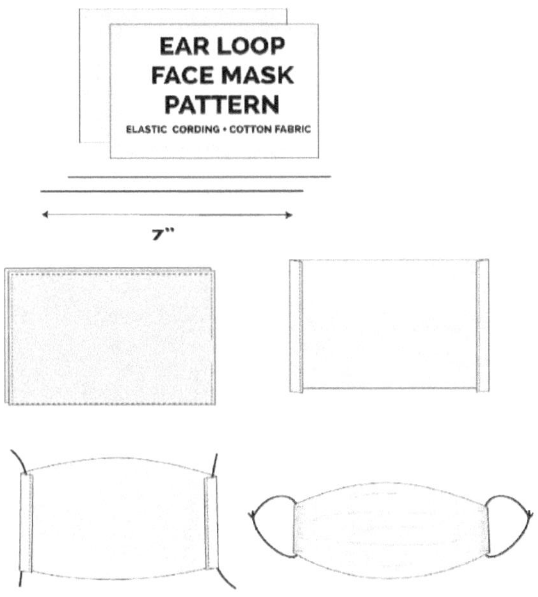

Latex-free face mask with tape binding (Bias)

No elastic is used in this type of face mask, and so it's a great option if you Do not have any.

-quilting cotton fabric, high quality cloth is best

–double fold 1/2" bias tape (or handmade
binding), two 35" strips

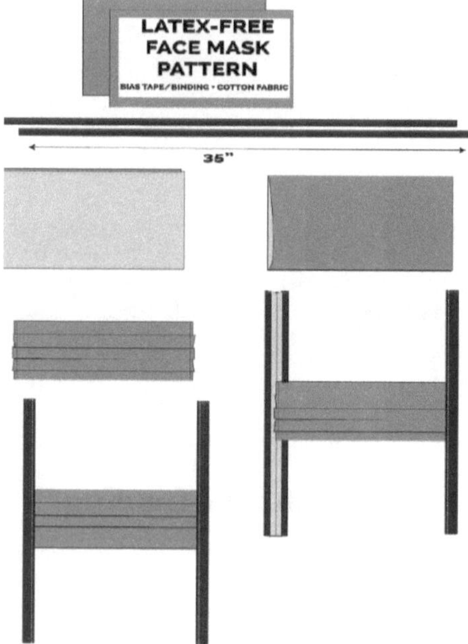

- Sew two squares aligning the top and
  bottom edge, leaving the sides open.
  Turn and press well.
- Pleat cotton fabric according to the
  pattern piece

- Enclose raw side edges with the middle of your bias tape strip.

- Sew bias tape together to sandwich mask in the middle.

- Tie ends of bias tape in small knots.

Sew and No Sew Instructions

Sewn Cloth Face Covering

Materials

- Two 10"x6" rectangles of cotton fabric

- Two 6" pieces of elastic (or rubber bands, string, cloth strips, or hair ties)

- Needle and thread (or bobby pin)

- Scissors

- Sewing machine

- Cut out two 10-by-6-inch rectangles of cotton fabric. Use tightly woven cotton, such as quilting fabric or cotton sheets. T-shirt fabric will work in a pinch. Stack the two rectangles; you will sew the mask as if it was a single piece of fabric.

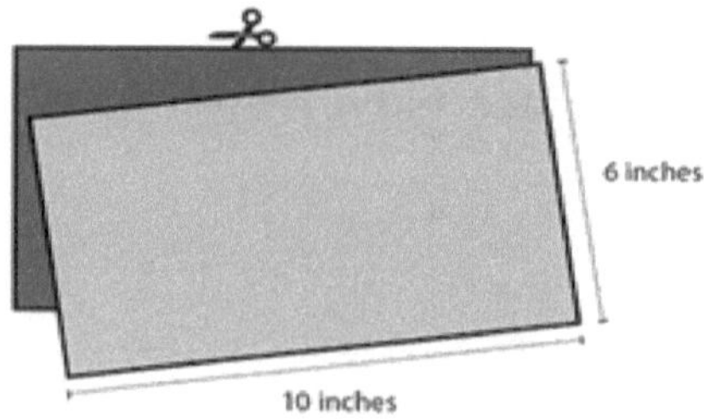

- Fold over the long sides ¼ inch and hem. Then fold the double layer of fabric over ½ inch along the short sides and stitch down.

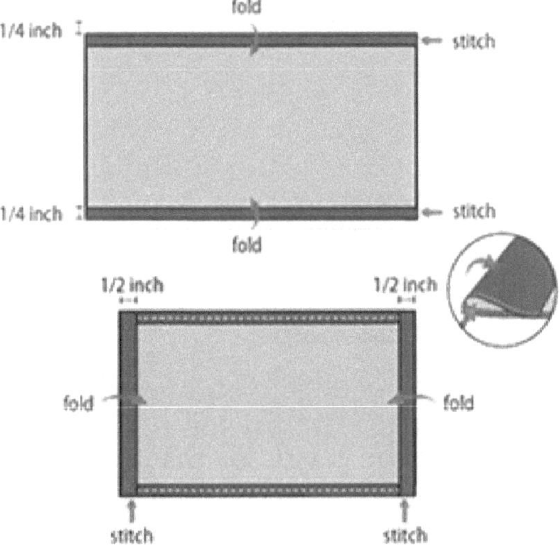

- Run an elastic band of about a 6-inch length of 1/8-inch wide through the wider hem on each side of the mask. These will be the ear loops. Use a needle or a bobby pin to thread it through. Tie the ends tightly.

If you do not have an elastic band, try hair ties or elastic headbands. If you only have a string, you can make the

ties longer and tie the mask behind
your head.

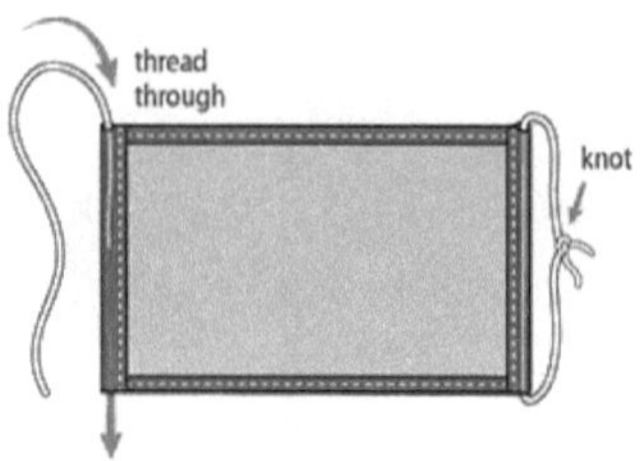

- Gently pull the elastic so that knots
  are tucked inside the hem. Align the
  elastic band on the sides of the mask
  and adjust, so the mask fits your face.
  Then secure the elastic band and
  stitch in place to keep it from slipping.

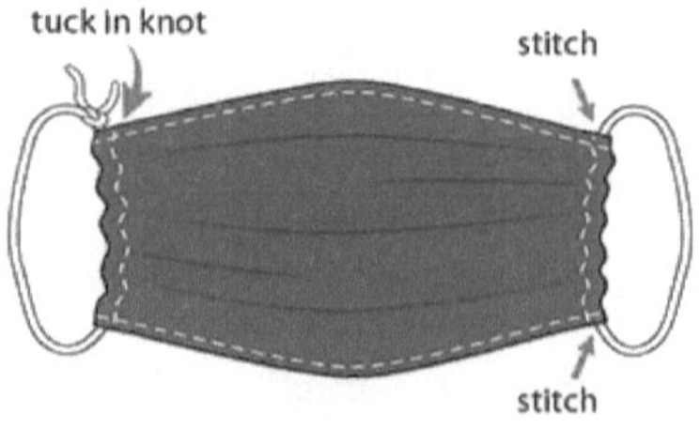

Quick Cut T-shirt Face Covering (no-sew method)

Materials

- T-shirt
- Scissors

Instruction

1.

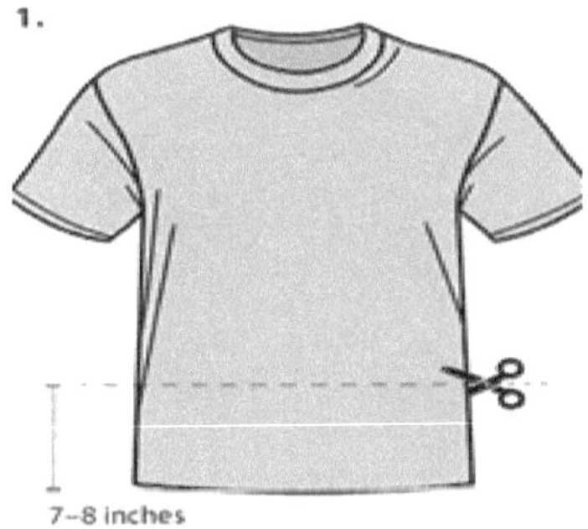

2.

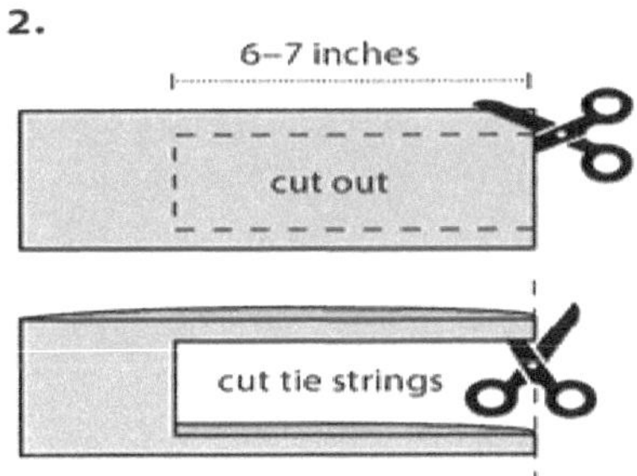

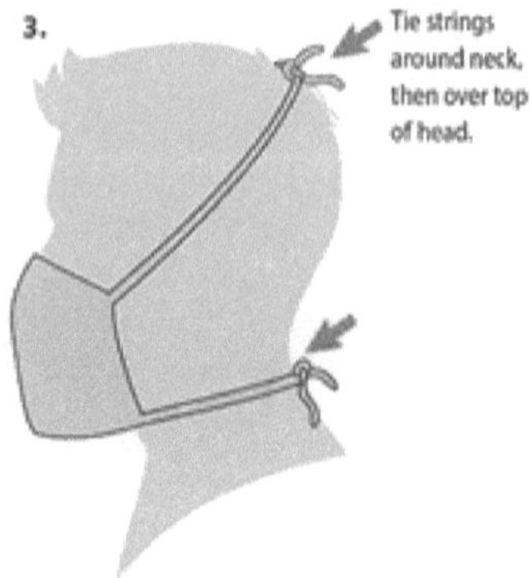

Bandana Face Covering (no-sew method)

Material

- Bandana or a square-shaped cotton cloth approximately 20"x20."
- Rubber bands or hair ties
- Scissors

Instruction

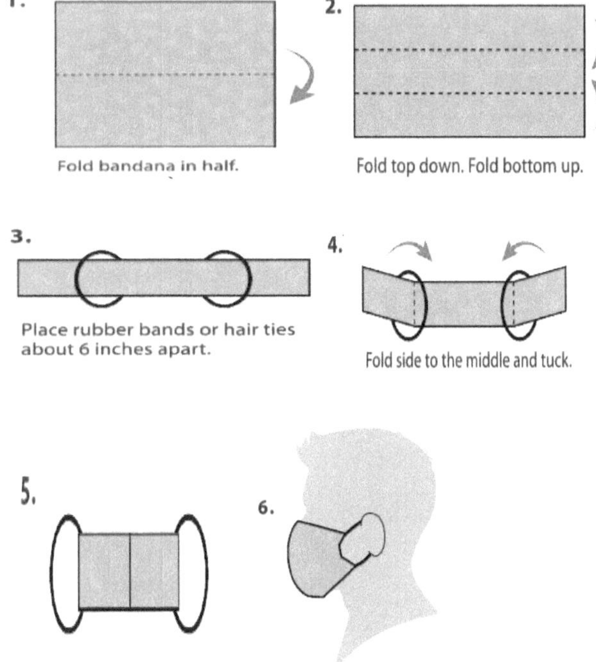

Reversible Germ-free face mask

The Germ-free Face Mask includes sizes:

- From 3-6 yrs. Allow up to 4inch distance from the nose bridge to the chin.

- 6-10 yrs. Allow up to 4.5 inches from the nose bridge to the chin.

- 10-14 yrs. Allow 5 inches from the nose bridge to the chin.

- Average adult. Up to 5.5inch from nose bridge to the chin.

- XL adult. Up to 6inch from nose bridge to the chin.

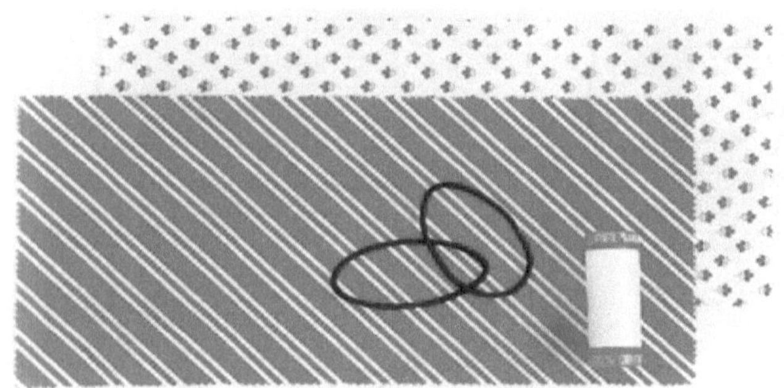

Material

- 2 Jolly Bar rectangles (5" X 10")
- 2 Elastic Hair ties
- Coordinating Thread
- Scissors

- Point turner

- Fold under 1/8" lengthwise on inner and outer fabrics
- Stitch the top

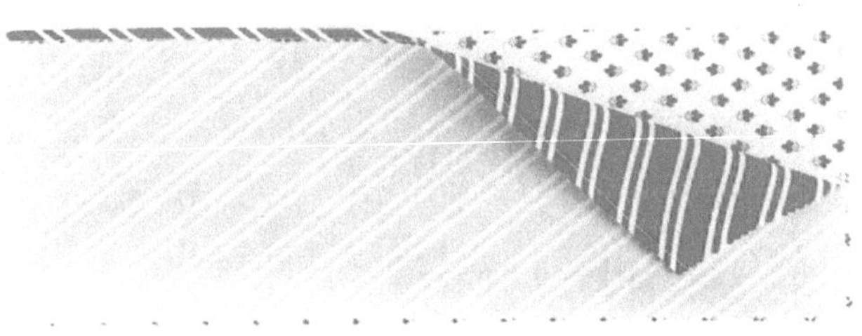

- Place fabrics right sides together.

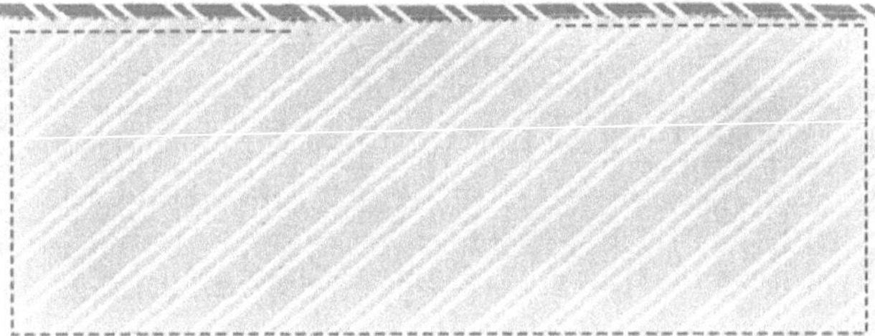

- Stitch using ¼" seam allowance around all edges

- Leave a 3" opening along the top (backstitch)

- Trim the four corners to the stitched to remove bulk

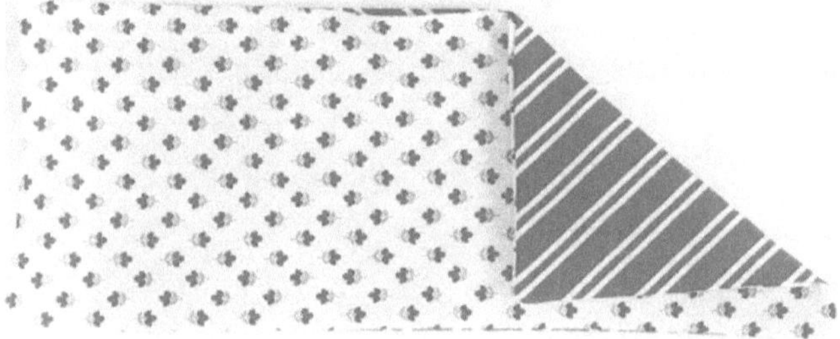

- Flip mask inside out and press well with iron

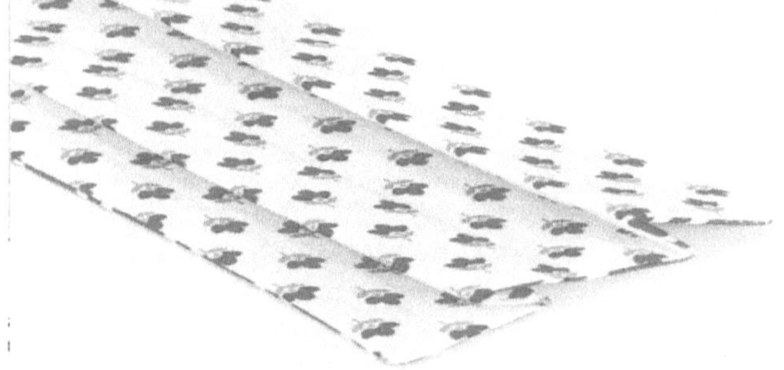

- Make pleats by folding mask in a zig-zag pattern every ¾" and press with an iron.

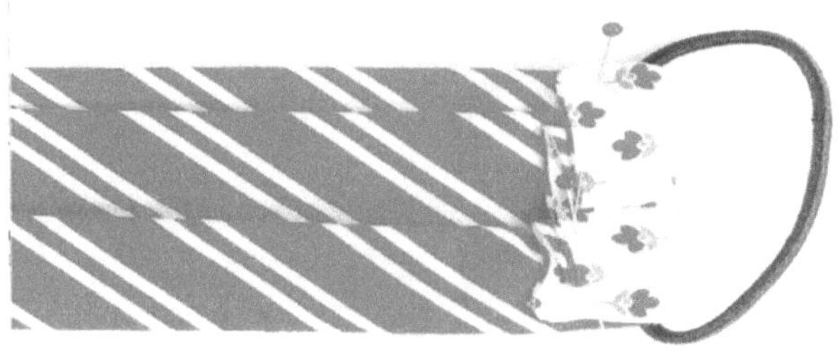

- Insert elastic hair tie and pin in place
- Topstitch making sure to avoid the hair tie

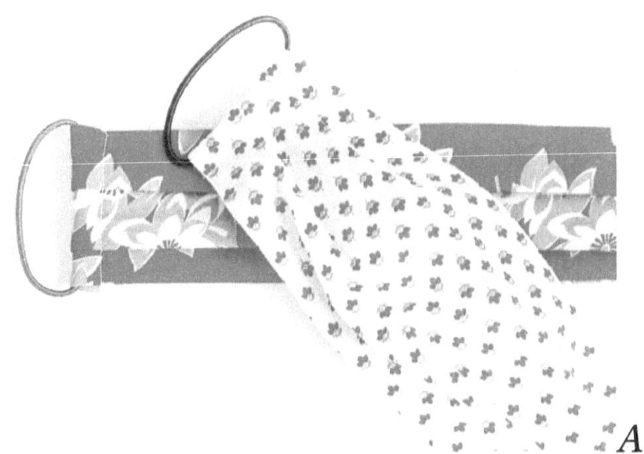

nd We are Done

DIY FACE MASK WITHOUT ELASTIC

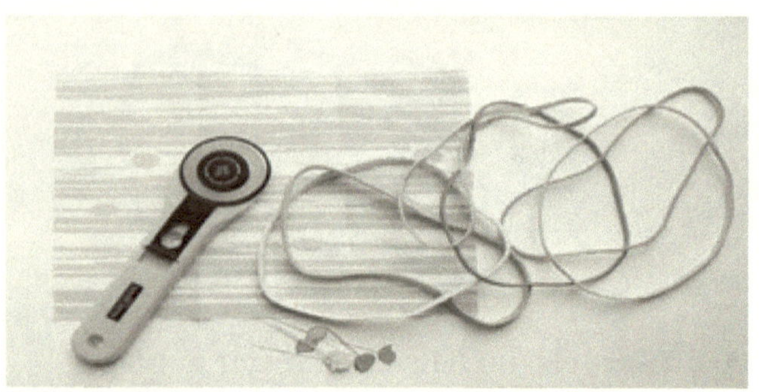

Materials

- Fabric – 2 rectangles per mask
- Elastic Headbands or Ponytail Holders
- Sewing Pins
- Rotary Cutter or Scissors
- Thread
- Ruler
- PDF Printable of Pattern

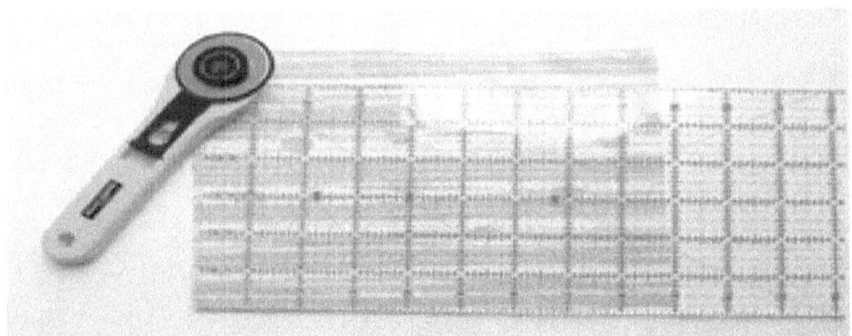

- Cut two rectangles shape with the size of the mask you want to produce - 7" by 9" for a medium-sized face mask and 7" by 10.5" for large-sized mask

- Cut elastic band into two parts according to the lengths required to work with. 5.5" - 6" for medium-

sized face mask and 6.5" for large-
sized mask

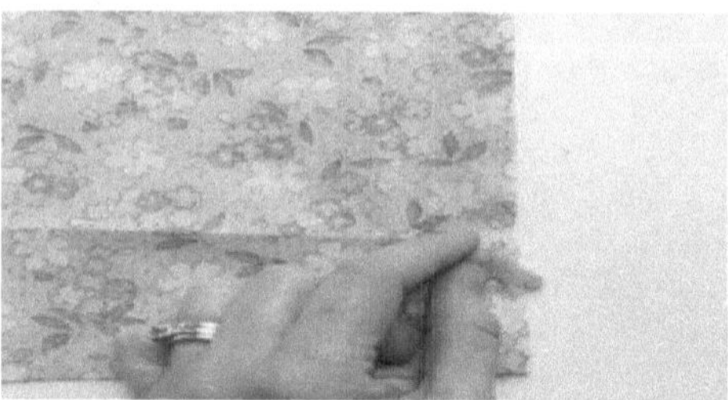

- Put the fabric, right sides together.
  Sandwich the elastic band along the
  shorter edges.

- Do not put the elastic to the corner of
  the fabric as it makes it more
  challenging sewing later. Let the
  elastic band be 1/2 inch away from
  the edge and sewing pin.

- Place the alternate side of the elastic
  and place at the opposite top corner
  and fasten pin. This makes the elastic
  sandwiched in between the two pieces

of fabric. Repeat this step on the
other side.

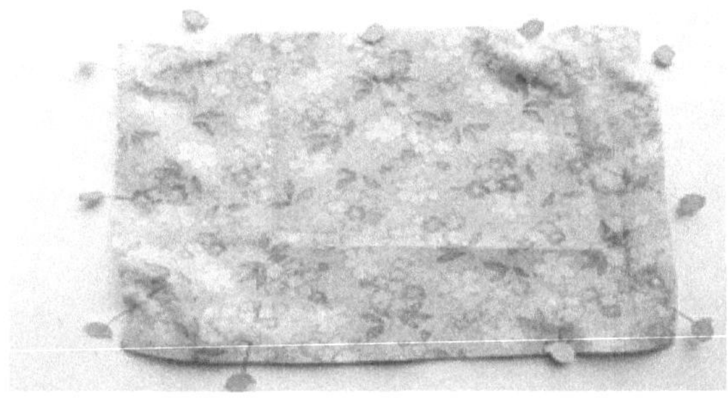

- Put in the rest of the fabric together.
- Sew around the edges of the rectangle

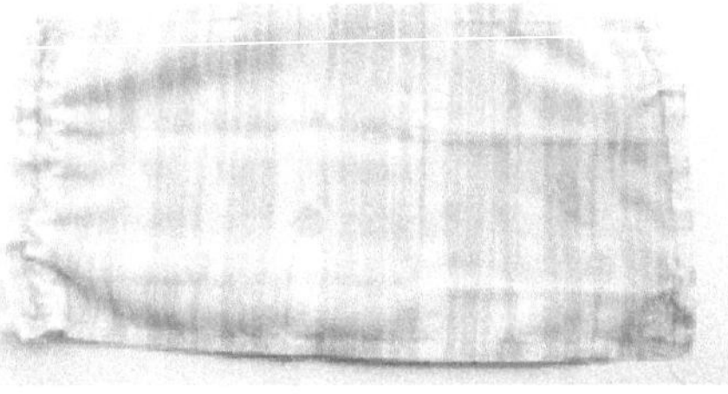

- pieces, leaving a 2-inch sized opening
  along one part of the more extended
  parts.

You can choose to make the seam big or small according to your preference. Sew around the elastic band a few more times to ensure the seam is keen to hold the fabric.

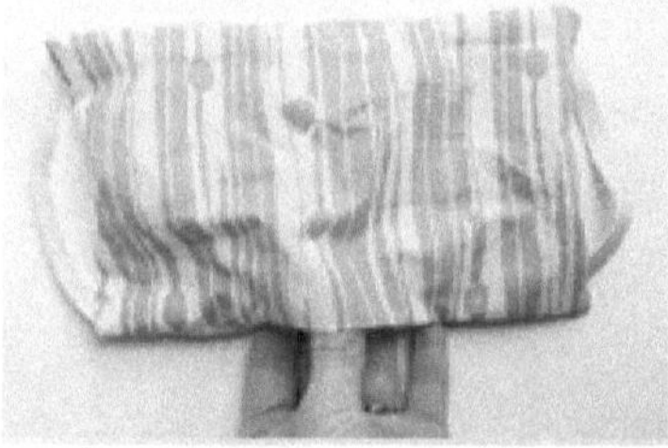

- Turn the mask right sides out.
- Poke out corners of the mask with a pencil or pointed objects.

- Stitch opening together.

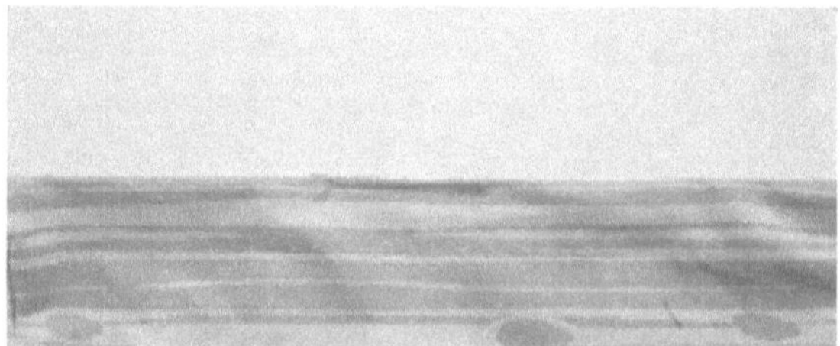

- Create two pleats along the shorter
  ends of the mask.

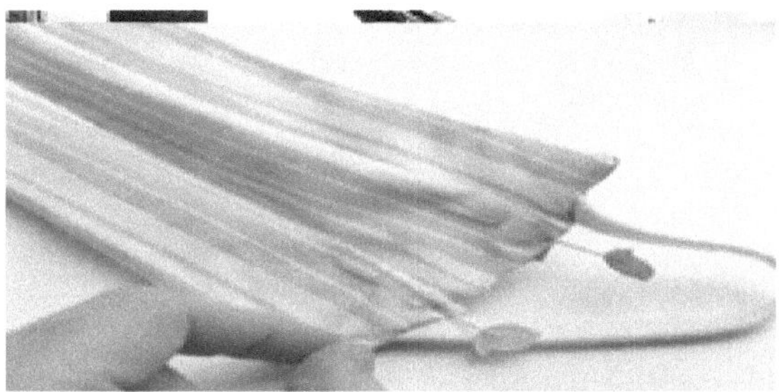

- The pleats do not have to be exact,
  but you want to fold the fabric and
  pin to create two pleats.

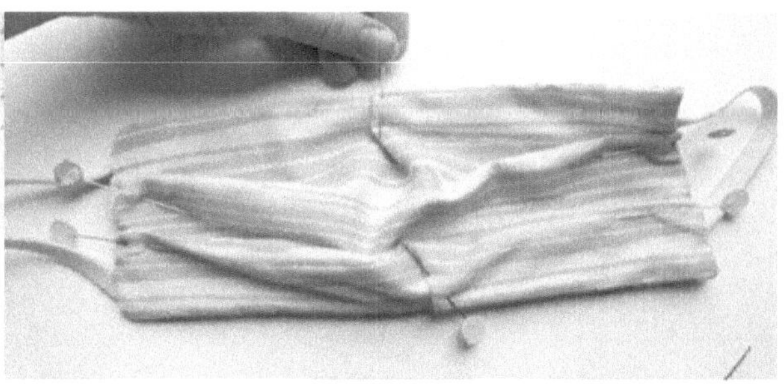

- Then make two little pleats along top
  and bottom sides of the mask. The

small pleats allow the mask to fit
more snugly around the chin and
nose.

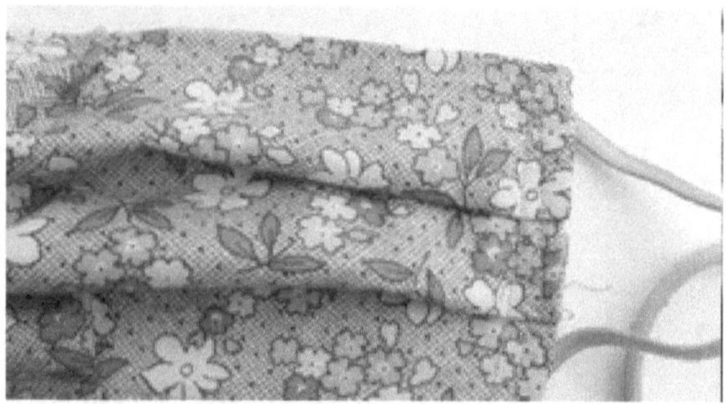

- Topstitch twice around sides of the
  mask.

You will want to topstitch at least two times
to make sure the seams are strong.

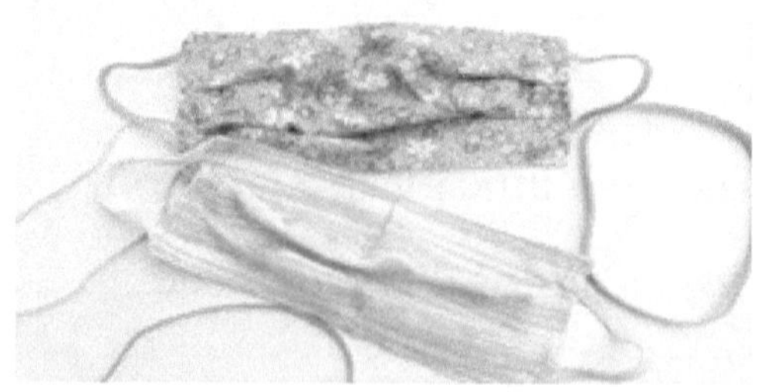

- Cut off the unwanted threads, and you are done.

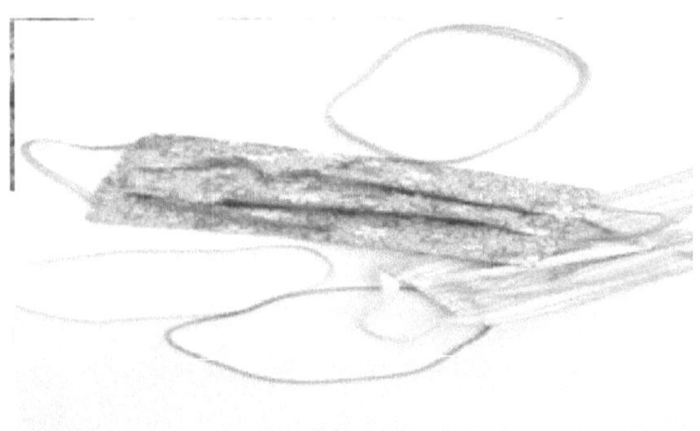

- Sanitize your hands or wash with a soap and clean water before putting on and removing a face mask
- Conscious care should be taken not to contaminate the inside of the mask and do not let mask rest on your chin
- Practice good health hygiene as best as you can!
- Any type of masks (N95, , fabric) should not be worn for too long. When

it gets damp, you should replace it. So, if you're sweating a lot, prepare replacement masks.

DIY Washable and reusable Face Mask in 12 Easy Steps

Material

- Two pieces of 6 inch by 9-inch fabric
- a 6" x 9" piece of iron-on interfacing (optional)
- Two pieces of ¼ inch elastic cut to 7" each

Instruction

- Cut out two pieces of fabric each measuring 6-inch x 9 inch.

- Cut out one piece measuring 6" x 9" for interfacing and press against the back of one fabric piece.

- Cut the elastic band into two pieces, with each measuring 7 inch.

- Place the two fabric right sides together.

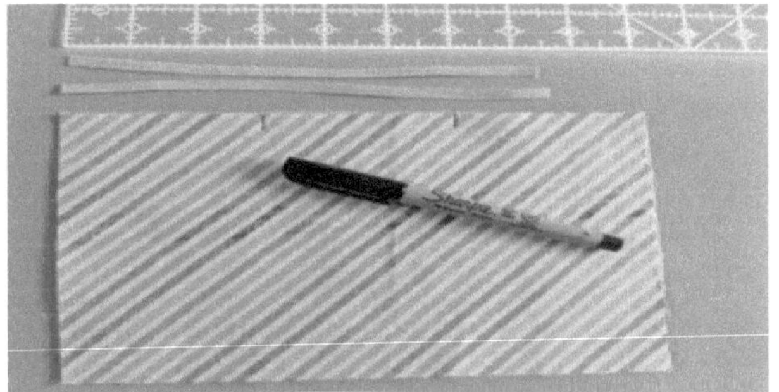

- Measure a 3-inch opening in the top so you can turn it right side out when you are finished sewing.

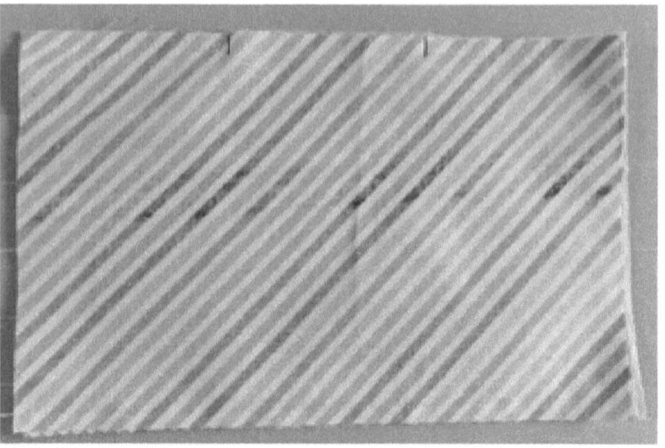

- Sew the top and bottom edges only.

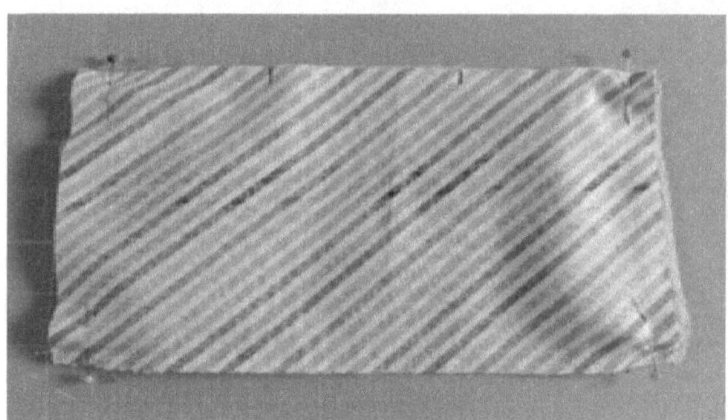

- Put the elastic inside the mask and pin it to the top and bottom of each side, keeping it fitted to the fabric. It should

be on the outside when you turn it
later.

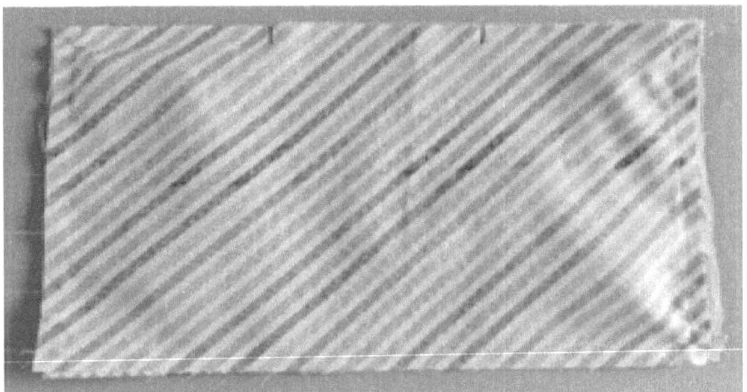

- Completely sew to clos each side and,
  back-stitch on the elastic.

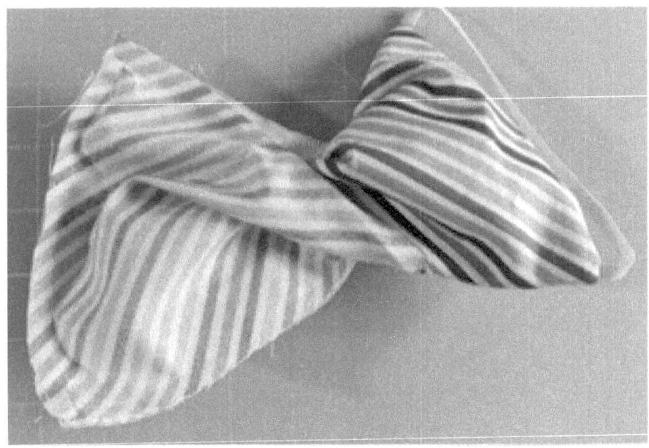

- From the hole created at the top, turn
  the mask right side out.

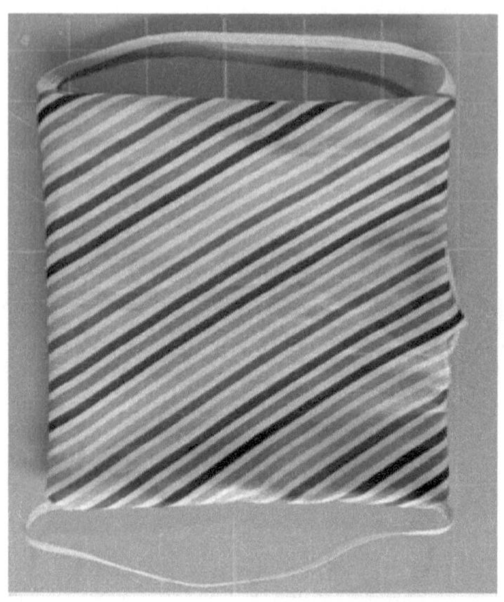

- Iron to make mask flat and add 2-3 pleats.

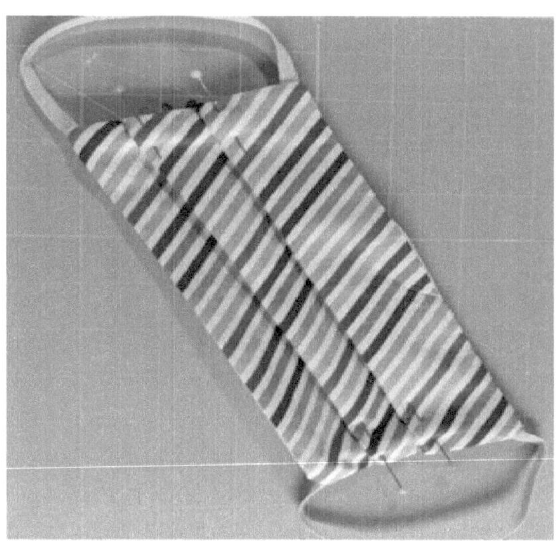

- Pin the pleats flat.

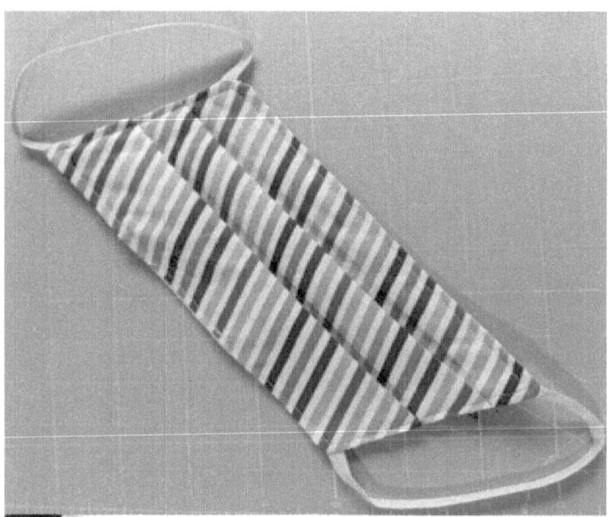

- Stitch round the edges of the mask for enclosure and to fix the pleats in position.

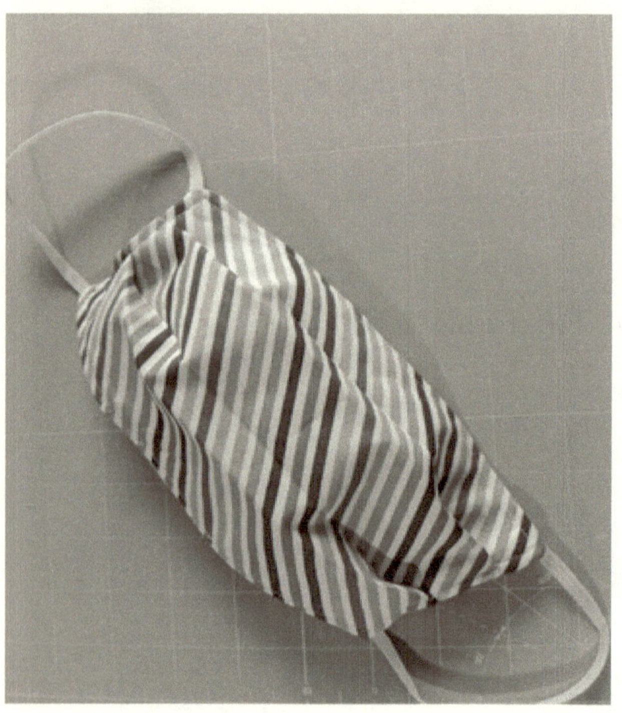

Mask is now ready for use. Wash and dry

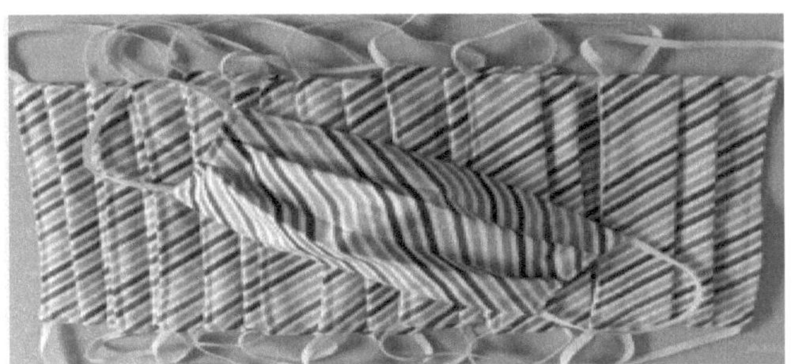

Important Tips:

- Use new fabric, and avoid vintage material that is tightly woven. Polyester or moisture-wicking fabric is an ideal substitute).

- You are allowed to finish the top edge of the fabric before stitching the mask together. Remember to create a small opening in the top so that a filter can be fitted into facemask.

- Attach ties to the mask if there is no elastic, so that it will be tied rather than being looped ears.

- Fabric face make are not substituted to N95 and are not very effective but they offer some level of protection

Making of **OLSON** Face mask pattern

Materials Needed

- Cotton Weave Fabric

- All-Purpose Thread

- 2 Hair Ties

- Scissors

- Doubled-Sided Skin Adhesive

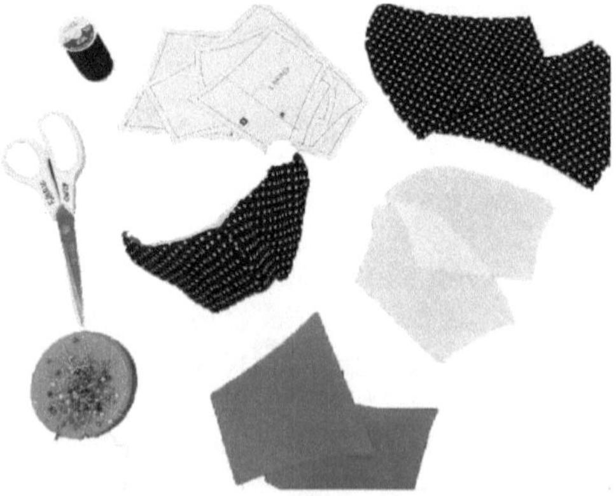

Hair ties and tapes with double sides will be applied at the hospital, to allow for different sizes

Instructions.

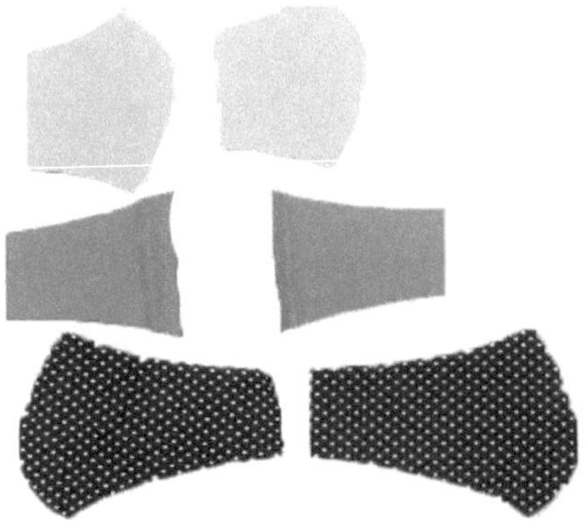

- Using the patterns above, cut one of each shape. You will need six pieces

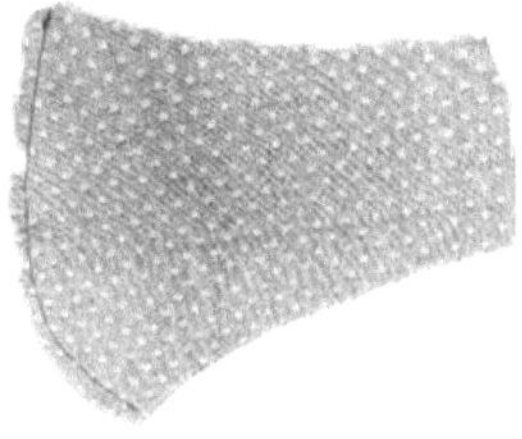

- Sew face one and face two together alongside 3

- Sew mouth 1 and mouth 2 together alongside 3.

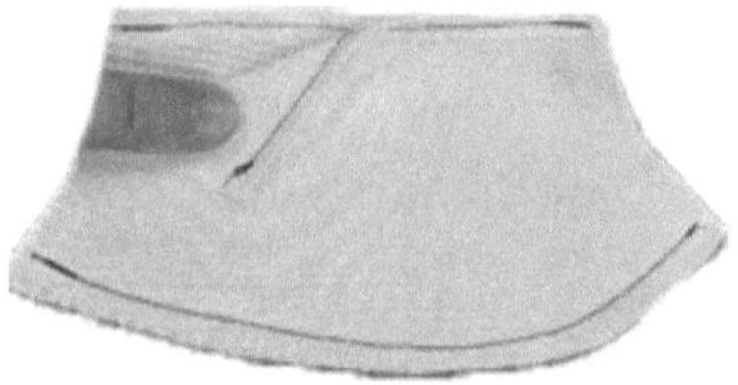

- Place side five over 1/4 inch on mouth 1 and mouth 2 and sew.

- On cheek one and cheek twofold side Six over 1/4 inch and sew down.

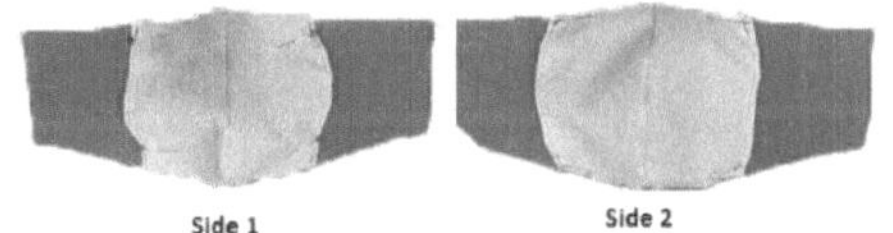

- Match cheek one and mouth one at the dotted line (7). Sew a 1-inch tack at side one and side two where the two pieces overlap.

- Repeat Step 6 for cheek two and mouth 2.

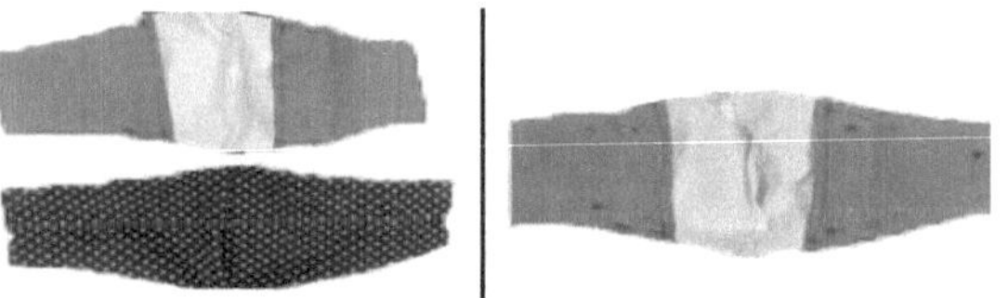

- Align the perimeter of the mask and sew with the fabric fronts facing each other.

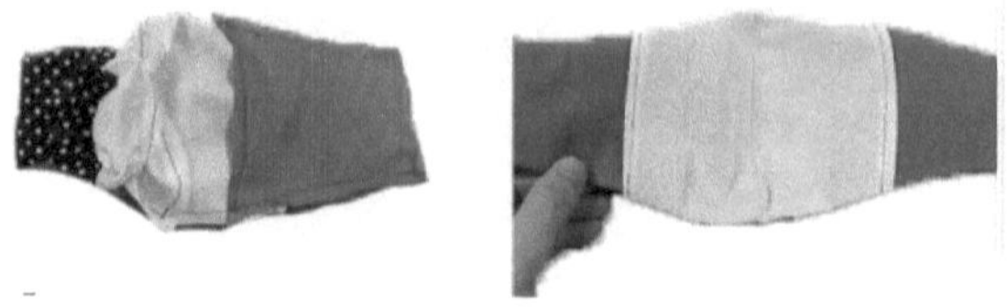

- Turn the mask right-side out using one of the slits between the mouth and the cheek.

- Fold the fabric on the end of the mask and insert the hair tie then sew.

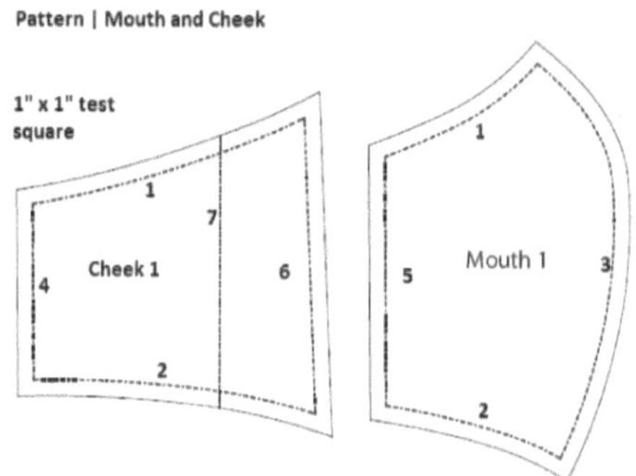

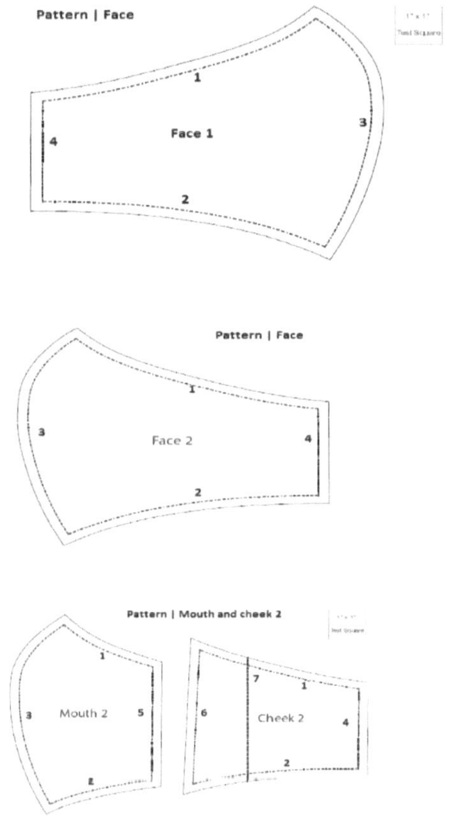

Making a Face Mask from Paper Towels

Materials

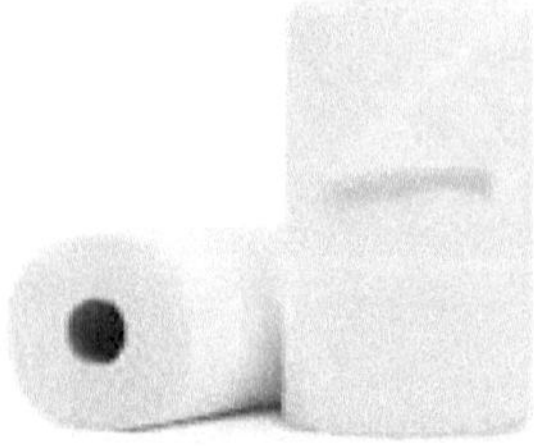

- Paper Towel with 6" perforations preferably we used Bounty paper towels or Blue Shop paper towels (they both have thick texture).

- Staples

- Rubber Bands

Instruction

- Rip off a sheet from the paper towel.

- Then, fold it about an inch, and fold another inch the other way.

- Continue process until entire sheet is folded.

- After you have repeated this process, take each end of the sheet, wrap around the rubber band, then staple it.

- On the perforated lines, fold paper towel in half. Make 3 tucks with the ends of about 1-1/2 inch in width. Fasten with a staple. repeat same process for both ends.

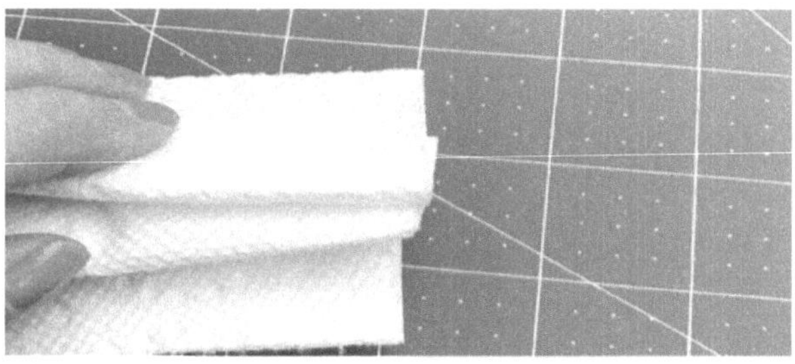

- Make 2 or 3 tucks and staple.

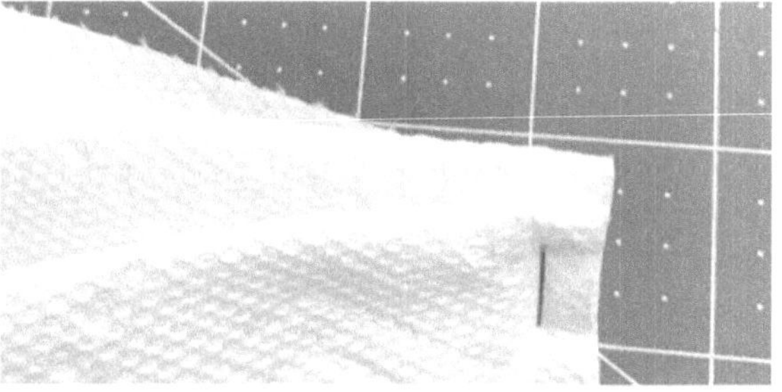

- Staple a rubber band of about 2-2/2-inch-long, to each end of the towel. Care should be taken not to staple through the rubber

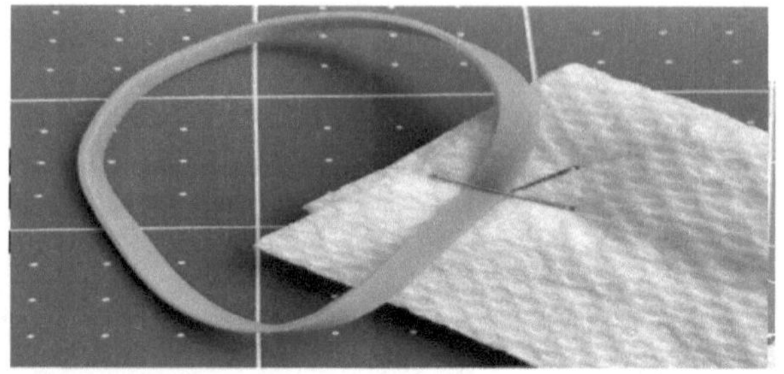

- Making Face Mask with Machine-
  Stitched Paper Towel

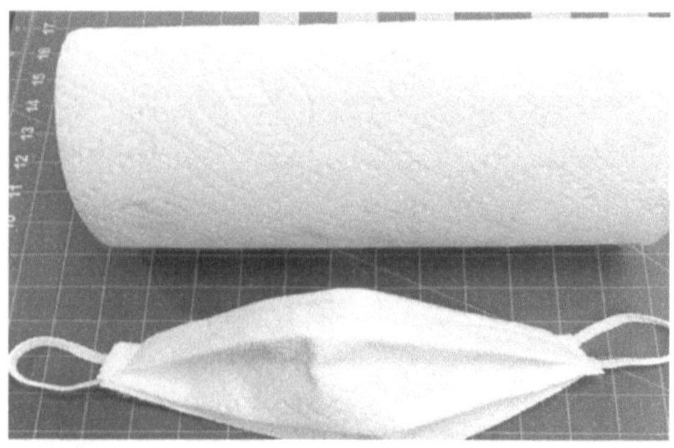

- Making this kind of face mask is time
  demanding. to make this mask, use
  Bounty perforated paper towels with a

chenille stem to shapen the mask to
fit the bridge of the nose.

- Fold paper on 6' perforation.
- Fold ½" to 5/8" from edge, stitch
  with chenille stem to fold.

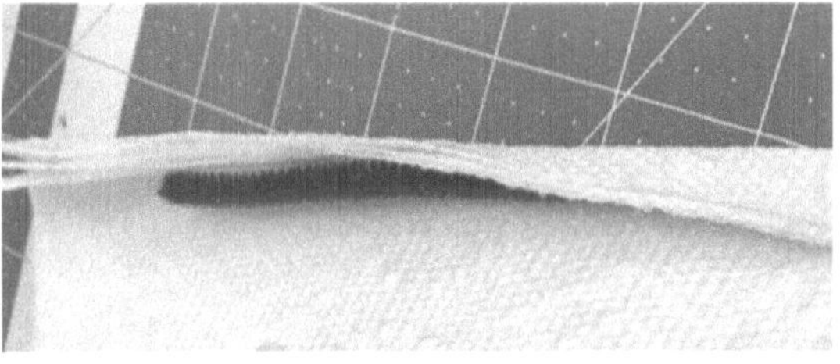

- Conscious care should be taken not to
  stitch directly on the chenille stem or

risk breaking a needle. Make 2-3 tucks in the mask and stitch the ends. Stitch a 5" piece of shoestring (or elastic if you have it) on the edges.

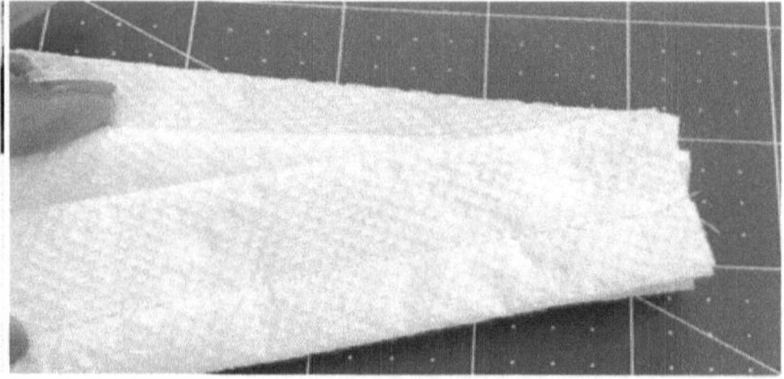

- Make 2-3 tucks and stitch
- Stitch shoelace to the edge

The length of the shoestring (or elastic) can always be adjusted in any size to fit your face.

Summary

CDC Recommended the use of Cloth Face mask by the General Public

N95 Respirators are not for Use by the General Public but for medical first responders and health care workers.

masks are not designed for use only once. Safely remove and discard face mask if it is damaged, soiled, damp or breathing is becoming perplexed. Replace with a new mask. Discard mask safely in a plastic bag or trash bin, wash your hands immediately after handling a mask.

N95 respirators and /face masks (face masks) are classified as personal protective equipment. They protect the user from inhaling or ingesting airborne particles and liquid contaminating the face

People suffering from chronic respiratory, cardiac, or other medical respiratory conditions should contact their healthcare specialist before using an N95 respirator because the N95 respirator can make it more difficult for the wearer to breathe. Some models have exhalation valves that can make breathing out more comfortable and help reduce heat build-up. Note that N95 respirators with exhalation valves should not be used when sterile conditions are needed.

Always protect yourself by using a face mask to cover mouth and nose when in a public environment.

Acute respiratory diseases can be spread by you to others, even if you do not feel sick.

Everyone should wear a cloth face cover or face mask when they have to go out in public.

Face mask coverings should not be used on children less than 2 years, anyone with breathing difficulty, or unconscious, incapacitated, or otherwise unable to remove the mask without assistance.

The cloth face mask is for the protection of other people from you supposing you are infected.

Do NOT use a facemask specifically
designed for first responders and health-care
workers.